Secrets of wa

By Bhaskar Mishra

Text Copyright © 2018 Bhaskar Mishra

All rights reserved

Table of contents

Introduction

Why water cure

Role of water in the body

Benefits of drinking water

Water can be a poison

Your body may throw out the water in place of assimilating it

When and how much water to drink

RO water may not be good for your body

Does intake of tea, coffee, juices, soft drink, cold drink etc qualify as water intake?

How Alcohol kills you?

How to tell your body to use water efficiently

Advanced methods of water cure

Water cure for various diseases

- Asthma
- Acidity, acid reflux, heart burn and indigestion
- Acne
- Constipation
- Diabetes
- Cardiovascular and Heart diseases
- Arthritis, joint pain, knee pain and back pain
- Skin diseases: get healthy glowing skin naturally
- Obesity: get clearly discernible results within four weeks
- Erectile Dysfunction
- Kidney stone and Kidney pain

- Scaly and dried lips
- Hair fall
- Headache
- Sinusitis/Rhinitis

Legal notice

All rights reserved. No part of this publication may be copied, reproduced or transmitted in any form or by any means including electronic, mechanical, photocopying, recording etc without prior written permission of the author.

Disclaimer

This book doesn't substitute medical advice. Please consult a qualified doctor if you have any medical condition before following any advice given in this book. However, all precautions have been made to provide you the authentic and safe information author will not be responsible for any problem that may occur to you due to following any advice in this book.

Introduction

Have you read a number of books on water cure and after reading those books decided to drink more water, but most of the water you drank came out in the form of urine and you didn't get any benefit? Have your efforts to cure yourself through water not bore any fruit? If answers to these questions are yes then this book is exactly for you.

Actually any additional amount of water taken by you can be thrown out by the body. There is a secret to prevent body from doing so. All those books have not told you these secrets. There are secrets to ensure proper assimilation and use of water by the body. This book will teach you exactly this. After reading this book you will be able to reap full benefits of drinking water. Water will be properly used by the body and you will be able to get healthy glowing skin, fluffy lustrous hair and a fit & healthy body.

Did you know that water can be poison even? Did you know that RO water may not be as good as you think? Did you know that besides drinking, water may help you in other ways also in detoxifying your body?

Water cure is the need of the hour. Conventional system of medicine is not curing you, it is making you more ill. This statement has been substantiated under the chapter 'why water cure'.

After reading this book you will be better equipped to use water for detoxifying your body. By practising the techniques of water cure in this book you will get a lighter & healthier body as well as a sharper and calmer mind.

In the second part of the book water cure protocols for a number of diseases (Asthma, acne, arthritis, acidity, acid reflux, indigestion, constipation, obesity, skin diseases, Kidney pain, erectile dysfunction, hairfall, headache, sinusitis etc) have been given.

Why water cure

Despite knowing so much about significance of water and its role in keeping you healthy, almost every one of us are skeptical about possibility of using water for curing various diseases. You should shed this reservation against water. Water cure is very effective in treatment of a number of health problems including Asthma, Arthritis, Kidney pain etc. Besides, there are a number of other reasons also for which you should adopt water cure methods.

I am enumerating some of them.

It is truly natural

The word 'natural' has become very fancy today. For a number of items this word is being used. Almost every product in the market claims to be natural. But are they? What is natural? On one extreme, anything that exists in the universe is natural. Had they not been natural, they could not have existed. On the other extreme, every thing that you inject from outside into your body is un-natural. In between is the opinion that those things which have been made by nature are natural and everything that has been made by man is unnatural. Even if we follow the middle path, are so called herbal or ayurvedic medicines natural? No doubt they have been made from naturally occurring substances, but have they been made by nature? No, a definite no. They have been made by humans. Proportions of various ingredients have been decided by man. So they cannot be termed natural. What if the person making them has not used right proportions of ingredients? What if computer program used to automate the process of preparation of these medicines were faulty? If we consider the parameter that everything made by nature is natural then we have a problem. We have the example of poisons. A number of deadly poisons have been made by nature both in animal as well as plant kingdom. They are definitely natural. They have been made by nature. All the proportions of ingredients in them have been decided by god himself. But, are they beneficial to us? No, a definite no. So, a natural inference is that everything that is even truly natural cannot be beneficial for us. So, we need to find only those natural things which are beneficial for us. For example, coconut water, fruits, nuts etc. All these have been made by nature. All ingredients have been put in them directly by god in right proportions for us. They are also beneficial for us.

Water is the most abundant, natural and naturally occurring substance on earth. Life originated in water. We are more than 70% water. So nothing else can be more natural and beneficial for us than water.

Conventional medicines don't cure you : they are making you more ill

Biggest reason for using water cure is that conventional system of medicine that we are using today is not curing us. It is just relieving us from some uneasiness, that too temporarily. If it gives relief in one symptom, after a period of time it creates another problem. Name one conventional system of medicine, which doesn't have any side effect. You can't name even one. Every medicine used in conventional system of medicine has side effects. They are not curing, they are just creating an illusion of cure. If you get any chronic disease and visit a doctor of conventional system of medicine, he will definitely give relief in symptoms of your disease for a while, may be for a year or two. But after that even if the problem for which you contacted the doctor appears to be cured, some other problem, probably more serious than the previous one, will appear. I shall give example of Arthritis. Arthritis has taken the form of an epidemic today. Almost everyone is suffering from one or the other problem of arthritis in his old age, even some younger ones. They visit doctors of conventional system of medicine. Doctors give them pain killers (steroid or non steroid based), calcium supplements and invariably a medicine to protect their gastrointestinal tract. The medicine for protecting gastrointestinal tract has to be given because these medicines can adversely affect intestinal mucosa. These medicines (given to protect gastrointestinal tract) too have their own side effects. Initially they relieve from the acidity but later on they cause more severe problems related with digestion. For the time being ignore side effects of these anta-acids. Move to two years ahead. Down the line two years of treatment what happens? Patient has three problems, one related with digestion, second related with cardio vascular system and third related with kidneys. Calcium supplements have formed plaques in arteries, which has caused high blood pressure and heart problems. Pain killers have adversely affected Kidneys. Now the patient has to visit at least three doctors, Gastroenterologist for problems related with digestion, Nephrologist for problems related with Kidneys and a Heart specialist for problems related with heart and Cardio vascular system. Biggest problem and irony is that Gastroenterologist will not bother for any side effect on Kidneys or heart, Heart specialist will not bother for any side effect on stomach or Kidneys and Nephrologist will not bother for any side effect on Heart or stomach. Have you actually been treated? I think you have not been treated, you have been robbed of your money, time and health during these two years, in the name of treatment.

Similar is the case with herniated disc. Generally your body corrects it on its own, but if for some or the other reason your body fails to do so then any conventional system of medicine don't work and doctors suggest surgery. Even after surgery, generally problems return after about 6 months or a year. Then one more surgery and then one more, you are trapped in a vicious circle.

(Fortunately there is a natural way to cure your herniated disc. Do read my book 'How to get rid of Sciatica and lower back pain without exercises'. In this book I have given a completely natural technique through which herniated disc gets cured. I myself have faced this problem and cured myself through this technique.)

No doubt in some cases especially acute ones and emergency ones, there is no option but to resort to conventional system of medicine. But in all other cases you should avoid it.

Ayurvedic medicines and even Homeopathic medicines can create imbalances in your body which may be difficult to treat and handle.

Water cure is free from any such problem. It cures in the gentlest possible way and is completely free from any side effect. Instead it has many benefits. If you are using water cure for your heart disease, it will also improve your digestion, liver, kidneys, skin and even hairs. This can be termed true cure.

It cures almost all diseases

There is not even a single disease in which water cure may not help you. In almost all diseases, it can help you and cure you. No doubt, it may take time but it is worth it.

It is dirt cheap

Economic aspect of treatment cannot be neglected. Treatment has become so expensive in some countries including USA that if you don't have health insurance you cannot even think of being treated. You can become penniless in the course of your treatment.

Water is freely available everywhere and you can use it wisely to cure almost all diseases.

Role of water in the body

Water has many unique properties. It is a very good solvent, it is bipolar in nature and it gets warm and cold slowly. Due to these unique properties water plays a variety of roles in the body. Not only in our body but due to these very reasons only, water is used in almost all factories.

Now let us discuss various roles played by water in our body.

Helps in digestion

Digestion is nothing else but breaking down of constituent of your food into smaller particles which can be easily absorbed by the body. The moment water comes in contact with food items it breaks down a number of its constituents into smaller particles through a process called hydrolysis. Water is bipolar in nature. Once any molecule which has ionic bond to bond its constituents, comes into contact with water, it disintegrates into its constituent ions. For example, common salt that you eat daily. It is made up to one atom each of Sodium (Na) and Cholrine (Cl). Sodium and Chlorine atoms are bound together by ionic bond to form one molecule of Sodium Choloride (NaCl), which is known as common salt. The moment they come in contact with water, it breaks it down into Sodium and Chlorine ions. These ions are then used by the body in various physiological processes.

Helps in regulating temperature of the body

Specific heat of water is significantly high. This means that temperature of water both increases and decreases at a slower pace. This property makes water the best agent for maintaining constant temperature in any system. Our body also, uses water to maintain constant temperature in the body and regulate it. Whenever outside temperature is high, body releases water through skin pores which on evaporating cools down the body. Whenever outside temperature is low, body decreases its hydration level by throwing out water through urine. This frees the body from the burden of heating so much water upto the body temperature. This is why skin becomes dry and scaly in winter season.

Helps regulate blood pressure in the body

It is necessary for the body to maintain an optimum level of blood pressure, so that it may flow properly all through the body and also deliver nutrients to cellular level. Body does this by controlling the amount of water in blood.

Water constitutes the bulk of blood. By controlling the amount of water in blood, body controls the amount of blood flowing through its arteries and veins at any particular time. By controlling the amount of blood, body controls the blood pressure.

Acts as a medium of transport

Water is a very good solvent. It dissolves nutrients into it and then carries them to cellular level along with blood. It also carries away waste products along with it from cells and tissues, which are extracted and excreted by Kidneys and liver.

Provides suitable environment in which various enzymes may work

Two virtues of water make it a very good agent for providing suitable environment in which various enzymes. First it is bi-polar in nature, thus enables free movement of ions through it. Secondly, its temperature changes at a very slow pace. Constant temperature and free movement of ions are necessary for various enzymatic reactions to appear. Both these factors are ensured by water.

Maintains ph balance in the body

Maintaining ph value in body is very necessary. ph value is basically a measurement of acidity or alkalinity of a solution. A low ph value means high acidity and a high ph value means high alkalinity. Some enzymatic reactions occur in high ph environment eg digestion while most others occur in lightly alkaline medium. Our blood is slightly alkaline. Water plays crucial role in maintaining ph balance in the body. Wherever in the body ph value decreaes, body increases water content there and ph value rises to the desired level. For the process of digestion, body increases acidity in the stomach and lowers ph value here by secreting Hydrocholoric Acid (HCl). After digestion is completed in the stomach, ph value is restored by water and bicarbonate (alkaline) solution secreted by pancreas.

Benefits of drinking water

It is said that 'water is life'. Water is needed for a number of biochemical processes which are necessary for life. It is not for nothing that first life forms originated in water. It is not only necessary for evolution of life but also for sustaining it. This is why almost all great civilizations have evolved along river banks. Huge factories are also established on river banks. It is said that third world war will be fought for water. Water adds volume to our blood. Just by regulating the volume of water in the blood, brain maintains optimum blood pressure in the body. Whenever it feels that water is less in the blood it asks kidneys to extract less water from the blood and form less urine and whenever it detects that water is more in blood it asks kidneys to take out more water from the blood and make more urine. Thus volume of water in blood is maintained by brain through kidneys. Water in our body also works as a medium of transport. Through blood it delivers the nutrients to every cell of the body and takes out their wastes and carries them upto kidneys where they are taken out and excreted with urine. Whenever, availability of water in the body is decreased this necessary mechanism of nutrition and detoxification suffers. On one hand cells get less nutrient and on the other hand they have to live with the toxins which otherwise should have been taken away. Thus gradually diseases crop in. Though there are innumerable benefits of drinking water in proper amounts I am giving you top six reasons.

Decelerates aging process

Aging is nothing else but the result of gradual wear and tear of the body. Aging process has two important elements. One is accumulation of toxins in the body and second is decreased capacity of body to retain and use water efficiently. Every physiological process in our body creates one or the other waste. Body has its mechanism to throw them out. Although, this mechanism is very efficient, still a minuscule percentage of waste is left in the body. Over a period of time the amount of these accumulated wastes increase so much that they start impeding body's normal physiological processes and gradually our organs become less and less efficient. A day comes when they start failing one by one and we die in the process. Second aspect of aging is body's decreased capacity to retain and use water efficiently. When we age, our body gradually unlearns to retain and use water efficiently. Why this happens is not known. Apparently, there is some switch in our genetic code which is responsible for it. Low level of hydration for prolonged periods is a cause but not the only cause. However, if we keep our body optimally hydrated all the time this process can at least slowed down if not completely turned off.

Water cure helps in two ways. First it keeps the toxicity in the body at minimum possible level and secondly it prevents body from unlearning to use water efficiently. Both these effects of water cure, decelerates aging and help us remain young for longer period of time.

Gives healthy glowing skin naturally

Natural glow of skin come from their water content. Abundant water makes skin cells fluffy, lively, supple and adds glow to them. This glow is 'glow of health'. Skin is the outermost part of the body. Our brain allocates water to its various parts in a hierarchical order. Most important and necessary processes and body organs are allocated water on priority. This priority keeps on decreasing with decreasing significance. Brain needs water most. Actually brain is about 80% water. So it takes water first. Next in order of priorities, it allocates water to other organs like liver, intestines, stomach, kidneys, heart etc. Skin comes in the bottom part of the priority list of brain.

This is why whenever availability of water is decreased to the body first sufferer is skin. Skin cells become rough and dry. They start looking ugly. Actually skin cells suffer on two fronts. First it gets less water as it is in the bottom part of brains priority list and secondly as it forms outermost layer of the body, it constantly loses its water content through the process of evaporation. Water molecules in the outermost cells of the skin just evaporate into the atmosphere. The process is hastened when the air is dry. It steals moisture from the skin cells. This is why in winters your skin loses its lustre. Thus it is necessary to drink abundant amount of water daily so that your skin may get it abundantly despite being in bottom part of priority list of brain.

Gives lustrous, shiny and healthy hair

Hairs are basically dead cells. Thus they are lower than even skin in the priority list of brain for allocation of water. Thus, if you drink less water, hair will suffer even more. However, as hair are basically dead cells and are least connected with the body, body cannot demand water back from it once it has supplied it to them. So impact of drinking of less water will be less visible on visible parts of hairs, but with the less availability of water, it will be supplied in lesser quantity in newly forming parts of hairs i.e. its roots. Due to lesser supply of water and nutrients, hair roots will become weaker and thus will become more prone to fall. This is why deficiency in the water may induce rapid hairfall. On the contrary if our body gets abundant supply of water, it will keep on supplying abundant water to 'hair formation process' also and so not only hair roots will become strong and healthy but also every layer of hair formed will be healthy and glowing. In this way you will get a lustrous, healthy and glowing hair.

Saves from joint pain, back pain and arthritis etc

Water is an important constituent of synovial fluid which works as grease at the joints. If water content in the body decreases, body is compelled to decrease water content in synovial fluid so that water may be made available for more important processes and organs. Joints and synovial fluids just ensure proper mobility for us. For our brain, this mobility function is not as important as digestion, maintaining blood pressure, proper functioning of brain, kidneys, liver etc. If any of these processes is hampered, our life, our very existence will be threatened. Thus body compromises on this function of mobility and takes out water from synovial fluid and allocates them to more important processes and organs. Once water content in synovial fluid decreases, it becomes thicker and its lubricating capacity decreases. With the decreased lubricating capacity, wear and tear at joints increases and also it becomes more difficult to move them. Damage occurs at joints on another level also. With the decreased water content in the synovial fluid, cartilages at the joints become drier and harder. They too lose their capacity and are less able to provide cushioning to the bones. Cartilages play very crucial role in the movement of joints. Cartilages are found at the ends of bones and provide cushioning to the bones. When cartilages become harder and less supple, they become more prone to injuries. Any inflammation in cartilages may also cause joint pain. In a number of cases of arthritis, this is the main reason behind joint pain. Cartilages have another problem also. There is not any blood supply to cartilages. So for them recovery is difficult. Their recovery takes more time. Only way to ensure proper nutrition and safety of cartilages, is to keep them flooded with synovial fluid. Cartilages are also there in between two vertebrae, where they are called discs. However, in spine role of synovial fluid is played by cerebrospinal fluid, but the case is same. Once water content in cerebrospinal fluid decreases nutrition to these cartilages also decrease. They become harder and less supple. They become thinner also and more prone to injuries. Injuries or inflammation to cartilages of spine may cause pain in respective areas. When you drink sufficient water, there is abundant supply of water in the body. It in turn ensures proper supply of water for synovial fluid, cerebrospinal fluid and cartilages. So, cartilages remain well nourished and you remain free from joint pain, back pain and arthritis etc.

Ensures proper and optimum functioning of brain

Your brain is more than 80% water. Brain keeps itself in top priority for allocation of resources available to the body. At any moment, it alone consumes about 20% of the total energy supply in the body. It also consumes most of the oxygen supply to the body. Similarly, it needs water to keep itself alive. So, it allocates water to itself on priority. However, to keep the brain alive proper functioning of liver, intestines, kidneys, spleen etc is also necessary. So brain makes a compromise, it starts shutting some of its functions and allocates water to these organs and other important processes. Cognitive processes are the highest level of functioning of brain. Whenever water becomes scarce in the body cognitive functions suffer first. Vision is also a more energy consuming process of brain. So if circumstances further aggravate vision becomes blurred. If situation further worsens, brain may decide to go in sleep mode in order to decrease water use and allocate water to other important life sustaining processes. Once brain decides to go in sleep mode, one may faint and may become unconscious.

Ensures proper digestion

Almost all digestive enzymes are water soluble. You cannot imagine the process of digestion happening without water. This is why whole of digestive tract right from buccal cavity to large intestine are kept well hydrated by the body. If less water is available to the body acidity in your stomach may increase causing heart burn etc on regular intervals. If acidity becomes a regular phenomenon, then ulcers may be formed in your stomach. Water is even more necessary for digestion of fats. Actually the enzyme pancreatic lipase which digests fat is water soluble and you must be knowing that fat molecules are not soluble in water. In order to being digested they first need to be emulsified which function is performed by bile secreted by liver. For emulsification process large amount of water is needed. Once fat molecules are emulsified, pancreatic lipase in water digest them. If there is less water, water will not be available for emulsification of fat molecules and fat cannot be digested.

Water can be a poison

John is my neighbour. He has been suffering from constipation right since his teenage years. Recently he read an article on internet about benefits of drinking water. He was so much impressed with the article that he started drinking water more and more, but unfortunately it didn't help him getting rid of constipation. He thought that perhaps he was not drinking enough water. So he further increased the amount and frequency of drinking water. With increasing water intake his visit to urinals also increased. It started disturbing his day to day life. Whenever, he had to go outside, he had to locate a urinal first, where he could empty his bladder. His bladder was full almost all the time. One fine day, I learnt that he was admitted to a hospital and doctors told him that his kidneys were about to fail. Luckily he was taken to the hospital in time and his life was saved.

What happened with John can happen with anyone. No doubt we are 70 percent water by weight. Water is an essential element of our health. It has a number of health benefits. Internet is filled with articles telling you the benefits of taking water, but these articles don't tell you the whole truth. They tell you only one aspect. I know a gentleman who by just asking you to drink water has made millions. Water if not taken properly can be dangerous also. John is an example. Excess intake of water damaged his kidneys. Excess of anything is bad. Water is also not an exception.

Excess intake of water puts extra load on kidneys. After you drink water, it is assimilated and absorbed by the body. Once absorbed, it enters into blood stream. Along with blood it travels through the body upto cell and tissue level. It takes impurities and a number of other metabolic wastes from cells and tissues and along with blood reaches kidney. Kidney extracts excess water as well as wastes of cells and tissues from the blood and forms urine. If one drinks less water blood becomes more viscous and kidney has to work harder to purify it. As water content is less in the blood, brain asks the kidneys to extract less water from the blood and make lesser urine. Two things happen due to this instruction of the brain. First as kidneys extract less water from the blood and make less urine, urine becomes more concentrated. This more concentrated urine is more likely to cause stones in kidneys. Secondly, as kidneys extract less water from the blood, despite its remarkable efficiency some wastes are left in the blood (though the quantity is very less). When one drinks water in excess quantities, blood becomes significantly thinner and it's tonicity decreases. Due to decreased tonicity in place of supplying nutrients to cells and tissues it starts extracting them. Sensing it brain asks kidneys to extract more water from the blood. In response to the instruction of the brain kidneys start extracting more water from the blood so that tonicity of blood may return to normal level. Along with more water it also takes out some nutrients from the blood. Furthermore, as kidneys have to extract more water and make more urine, that too more frequently, it has to work harder. If load upon it increases beyond a certain limit it may fail. Thus, both excess and less intake of water are bad. One should take only as much water (or slightly more) as is needed for optimal function of kidneys. If one drinks 100 glass of water within an hour, he can die of kidney failure.

Your body may throw out the water in place of assimilating it

Your body is smarter than you think. Absorption and assimilation of water in our body is controlled by brain through a hormone called ADH (Anti Di-uretic Hormone). Whenever brain detects that there is more water in blood, it decreases the secretion of ADH which signals kidneys to extract more water from the blood and make more urine. This is why whenever you increase your water intake most of your increased water intake comes out of your body as urine and the very purpose of increasing water intake is defeated.

No doubt you have increased the water intake, but your body is not ready to assimilate and properly use this increased amount of water. You will have to give some time to your body to learn to use this increased amount of water. Also you will have to apply some trips and tricks so that your body uses water in better and more efficient ways.

More efficient and smart your body is in assimilating and using water optimally, younger you will look. In advanced ages capacity of our body to assimilate and use water decreases. With the decreasing water content in our body it's efficiency and capacity also decreases. If we can prevent our body from unlearning to use water properly we can live young for more years.

When and how much water to drink

Timing of your drinking water is very important. There are times when your body is more prepared to use the water you drink. Similarly, at some other occasions drinking water can be even harmful for you.

When to drink water

Best time to drink huge amounts of water is the morning. For all night long you have not drunk water. Your body is thirsty. Every organ is demanding water. They are just crying for water. This is exactly the right time to drink huge amount of water.

Just after waking up, drink as much water as you can drink in one go. Luke warm water is the best. Most of you can drink about 1.5 – 2 litres of water in one go at this time. This water will take a full round of your body and after about half an hour a portion of it will come out in the form of urine.

This ritual of drinking huge amount of water in the morning should be done even before brushing your teeth. Yoga scriptures say that the saliva in your mouth in the morning is very beneficial for your health. If you brush your teeth before drinking water you may not be able to get benefits of this magical potion (your own saliva). Actually, as per the yoga scriptures, there is a centre in upper portion of your palate from where every time 'amrit' (life force) is trickling. In normal circumstances, this falls in the fire place in your stomach and is burnt. While sleeping this process is halted. Most of the 'amrit' (life force) that has trickled from this centre is still in your mouth. If you drink water (even a glass) this amrit can be utilised by your body. It will gift you a very good health and sound body.

Another recommendation of yoga scriptures is to keep the water overnight in a copper vessel and drink this water in the morning. Actually copper has a purifying property; it can kill bad bacteria and promote the growth of good bacteria. Good bacteria can work wonders for your health. These help in digestion. A number of components of your cannot be digested by the body, these are digested by these bacteria and made available to the body for ready assimilation. These bacteria can also synthesize a number of vitamins which may be lacking in the food taken by you but are needed by the body like Vitamin D, K, E, A etc. Copper vessel has another benefit also. It reacts with various impurities in the water and extracts them from the water. After being kept in the copper vessel overnight water becomes more pure and healthy.

After the morning ritual of taking large amount of water you should take one glass of water (about 200 ml) every two hours. If you can't remember or don't want to do it, you should take one litre of luke warm water in day time and one litre luke warm water in evening. In summers you can replace luke warm water with water at room temperature. If you want you can add some cold water to it to cool it down a bit more, but you should never drink chilled water from the fridge.

Again, just before going to sleep you should take a glass of water (about 200 ml). It will keep you hydrated in your sleep. But you should keep in mind that if you drink more water at the time of going to bed, it may disturb your sleep. You may have to go to bathroom during night hours. We don't want it. So you should drink only that much water in the evening and before going to bed so that you don't have to wake up twice or thrice for using urinal in night. A sound sleep is as important as keeping you hydrated.

Why you should never drink chilled water from the fridge?

This chilled water adversely affects your health. This chilled water makes sudden temperature changes in the body and your body may have problems coping with it. Your body will immediately try to heat this water and bring it to body temperature so that it can be used. If body cannot cope with the sudden change in the temperature caused by the chilled water, you may fall ill. From acidity, nausea, vomiting, indigestion etc to high fever anything can happen to you. Have you ever observed what happens when you keep a glass full of chilled water in the room? Small droplets gather on outer walls of the glass. From where did these water droplets come? Chilled water has condensed nearby water vapour molecules into liquid water. Same thing happens in your lungs when you drink chilled water. When you inhale you inhale not only oxygen but also water vapour in the air. When this chilled water enters your throat and passes through trachea, it converts some of the water vapour in your inhaled air into water molecules, which directly reach your lungs. As long as the amount of water thus condensed by the chilled water is not much, there is not any problem. These water molecules will be re-converted into water vapour by the heat in your lungs and exhaled out. But, if more water molecules are formed or for some or the other reason your lung cannot exhale out these water molecules, these will accumulate in your lungs and adversely affect functioning of lungs. This situation is called 'oedema of lungs'. In this condition water is filled in lungs and lung is unable to throw it out. A number of people develop this condition just because of drinking chilled water from the fridge.

When not to drink water

You should not drink water just before and after taking meal. There should be at least a gap of 30 minutes before and after your meal. Actually, food that you eat is digested in the stomach by the Hydrochloric acid. If you take water just before or after or during taking meal, it will dilute the acid in your stomach and it will not be able to digest the food. Improper digestion of food items in stomach will cause a number of other problems like gas, acidity etc. If you can't avoid taking water during the meal you should try to take the least possible quantity, just as much as is dire necessary. By practise, very soon you will not need water during eating, most of the time.

RO water may not be good for your body

RO water is purified water which have been purified through the process of Reverse Osmosis. Waters purified in this manner can have no mineral content. In normal water a number of minerals are dissolved. These minerals have two roles. First it is needed by the body for various physiological processes. Secondly, these keep the tonicity of water at optimum level. Tonicity is the term used to compare the concentration of solutes in a solution. If concentration of solutes in a solution is more then it is called hypertonic and when concentration of solutes in a solution is less it is called hypotonic. Generally water flows from hypotonic solution to hypertonic solution in order to balance the tonicity. When you drink RO water, as it is devoid of mineral content, tonicity of blood decreases when it reaches blood stream. In order to keep the tonicity of blood at optimum level (which is necessary for delivery of nutrients to cell level) body mixes minerals and electrolytes into the blood from its reserves. Thus when you drink RO water, your body loses precious minerals and electrolytes in place of gaining it.

What is the way out

You don't need to worry much as most of the companies manufacturing RO water purification systems are smart enough to keep its setting at such level that some impurities still remains in the water purified by these systems. Some RO water purification systems, deliberately mix some impurities into the water after its purification so that its tonicity doesn't fall below a certain level. Some of them even leave it to you to choose what level of purification you want. Talk to your RO water purification system supplier about it. He may help you keep the settings of your RO system at healthiest level.

Mineral water is the best

Mineral waters taken from natural springs are the best. They contain optimal amount of minerals in them. Many companies sell them in the form of bottled water.

If you cannot get them or afford them, mix electrolytes in your drinking water at least once in a day or once in two days. You can procure them easily at any chemist shop. You can ask for ORS (Oral Rehydration Solution) from them. These are generally suggested to persons suffering from diarrhea. Talk to your doctor for best suitable frequency of taking it for you.

If you still can't get one or can't afford, just add about a tea spoon full of sugar (honey is the best) and one fourth tea spoon full of salt to one glass of water (about 200 ml) and drink it once a day. It should suffice to maintain good electrolyte balance in your body.

Be warned that if you are suffering from diabetes or high blood sugar, ORS or adding sugar or honey to water may be harmful for you. Before doing so talk to your doctor.

Does intake of tea, coffee, juices, soft drink, cold drink etc qualify as water intake?

Intake of tea, coffee, soft drink and cold drink don't qualify as water intake. In fact all of these are di-uretic and tell your body to lose water. Thus all of them cause dehydration in your body. You may be in the illusion that with tea, coffee, soft drink and cold drink you have taken water and have fulfilled your daily quota of water intake, but in reality you lose more water than you take with these drinks. So all of them are obvious 'no-no' as far as qualification on the parameter of water intake is concerned.

However, case with fruit juices is different. If it is pure and raw juice then it does qualify as the water intake but if it is processed and packaged juice then it cannot be counted as water intake. In fact in processed and packaged juices a number of preservatives are added so as to give them a longer shelf life. Additionally, high amount of sugar is also added. Sugar adds taste to the juice and also acts as a preservative. Due to these reasons they become diuretic in nature and cause fluid loss from the body in the form of urine. You obviously don't want it.

How Alcohol kills you?

Alcohol is absorbed by the body at a faster rate than water. It alters the normal functioning of your brain. In normal circumstances, whenever it detects that there is less water in the blood, it releases a hormone called anti-diuretic hormone (ADH) which instructs kidneys to absorb less water from the blood and make less urine. When alcohol affects brain it affects this process at two levels. First, it reduces the capacity of the brain to detect water content in the blood, so brain is unable to properly detect the amount of water in blood. Secondly, it inhibits brain from secreting anti-diuretic hormone (ADH). In the absence of ADH, kidneys extract more water from the blood and make more urine and you become dehydrated. The worst part is that as brain is unable to properly detect the water content in the blood even in the case of extreme dehydration it doesn't take any action. Your kidneys keep on making more urine and dehydrating you more. Result is that a number of organs of your body cannot work properly including your liver. Due to dehydration, acidity in your stomach as well as blood stream increases. This acidity further aggravates the problem. Increased acidity puts extra load on pancreas (pancreas make bi-carbonates to neutralise the extra acidity). This increased load on pancreas will eventually lead to diabetes. In the absence of less water, liver will also not function properly. As all the fat soluble wastes and toxins are treated by the liver, toxicity in the body will keep on increasing leading to more diseases.

Biggest problem with the alcohol is that even if you try to compensate water loss by drinking more water, your attempts will go in vain because in the absence of ADH, you will keep losing more water through urine than you drink.

Another problem with alcohol is its dependency syndrome; every time you need more alcohol to reach the same level of ecstasy (if there is one) that you reached last time. You are forced to take more alcohol and increase its intake. More alcohol means more dehydration.

Finally a day may come when you cannot live for a day without alcohol. Gradually, this habit of alcohol will create chronic dehydration in your body and you may die of multiple organ failure.

Moral of the story is 'leave alcohol' or at least decrease its use to bare minimum.

How to tell your body to use water efficiently

Before I move ahead I want to ask you a question. Whom would you allow to stay in your home? You have been given three choices. First one is friendly and warm, second one is aloof and cold and third one talks too much and is hot headed. I am sure every one of you will decide to keep the first one in your home. Simila is the case with water. First person as told above is like warm water, second one is cold water and third one is hot water. Your body loves the first one. It loves warm water. Like warm water is readily absorbed by the body. It travels whole body and reaches maximum number of cells delivers them nutrients and takes away the waste products from them, caries ths waste producte with it upto kidneys. And thus better cleans our body at the cell level. Do you know life was first formed on earth in a broth of mineral rich luke warm water? This fact should literally assure that 'luke warm water gives life'.

If water is cold, your body will have to heat it first before sending it to cells. It is an expensive process from energy point of view. In place of using this water your body may decide to expel most part of it agar the earliest and result of this decision of your body will result in coming out of this water as urine much earlier than expected.

Similarly if water is too hot it may damage internal mucosa.

Role of fiber (fibre)

Fibers are basically indigestible parts of our food. They are also known as roughage. They are such parts of plants which cannot be digested by our digestive system. As they are indigestible, fibers don't give our body nutrients or energy but they have a very interesting property i.e. they can absorb water molecules and trap them. This property of fibers is very useful for our body. Once digestible parts of our food are digested and absorbed in small intestine, indigested parts reach large intestine. Last stages of digestion occur here. Indigested food remains here for comparatively longer time. Actually the process of digestion (from mouth to anus) may take about 30-40 hours to complete. Food remains in your stomach and small intestine only for 6-8 hours, for remaining 24-30 hours it remains in large intestine. Large intestine's role is to absorb water from indigested food, make them solid and convert them into stool, so that they may be excreted out. If you intake more fiber, more of it will be there in large intestine. More fibers in large intestine means availability of more water for the body, as they trap water. If needed body can absorb the water trapped in these fibers through large intestine anytime. Thus they serve as secondary source of water for the body and it can remain hydrated for longer time. With ample fibers in your diet, your large intestine works like a water bank for your body. Your need to drink water more often is obviated. On the contrary, if fiber content in your food is less, less water will be available for the body through absorption from large intestine. So, you will need to drink water more often to keep yourself hydrated.

Good sources of fiber are whole grains, nuts, fruits, salads, vegetables (especially leafy ones) etc. As a general rule more processed a food item is less fiber will be in it. There is almost nil fiber in egg, fish and meat. Similar is the case with bread, pizza, pasta etc.

Role of exercise

The saying 'use it or lose it' goes well even for cells. If your cells need less water and at lesser intervals it will gradually unlearn using it properly and efficiently. Exercise reverses this process. If you are the one, who whenever increases his water intake, his visits to urinals increase and there is no benefit to the body, then you need to exercise. During exercise our body needs more energy. It's metabolic rate increases. Heat, at the cellular level, increases. Now cells need water to cool them down so that it may keep working efficiently. This need of water forces the cells to better use water. After you start exercising regularly within a month you will notice that your capacity to retain water in your body has increased. If you felt thirsty after exercising just for 15 minutes in initial phases of your starting exercising, after a month or so you will not feel thirsty even after exercising for an hour. This has happened because your body has learnt to better store and use water.

It is not at all necessary that you do rigorous exercise. It should be mild but not so mild that there is not load upon your body. Its intensity should be so that your heart rate increases slightly. Optimum level is that when you are panting but can still talk with someone.

Exercise at this level of intensity at least for 30 minutes every day. You can choose cycling or walking (with intermittent jogging) as a daily routine of exercise. Weight training is a good choice, but you should increase the weight only gradually. Don't let your ego come in your way. Start with mild weights.

Thus keys to teach your body to use water smartly are (i) taking luke warm water (ii) add more fibers in your diet and (iii) do regular exercise.

Advanced methods of water cure

Besides drinking there are a number of other ways also to use water for the benefit of body. Taking bath is also one such way. From the perspective of the body your skin is the outermost layer. When you drink water, it will come from inside out, thus it will take time to reach skin cells. It may not even reach in proper quantity. When you take bath or sprinkle water upon your body the whole process is reversed. Now skin cells are the first to get water. They get it directly and abundantly. Cells in the outermost layer of skin absorb this water directly. For this absorption of water by outer skin cells body doesn't need to spend any energy. It is the most energy efficient process of water absorption (just for outer skin cells). Furthermore, when you take bath and skin cells absorb this water, this is also an indication for the brain that water is abundantly available. It doesn't need to worry for the availability of water. If you can take bath with water then you must have enough water for drinking, brain thinks like this. Now brain directs all body organs to use water at will. There is no rationing on water from the side of brain. This is why bathing refreshes you.

Now I am telling you about some more advanced uses of water for purification and detoxification of the body.

Nasal irrigation

There is kriya in yoga which uses waer for purification of the body especailly sinuses. Sinuese play important and crucial roles in the process of respiration. While inhaling air passes through nasal sinuses where these are moistend by the water in the mucus in sinuses. If inhaled air is dry it may rob the moisture from throat and lungs and you may fall in severe problem. However, at times blockages, inflammation and infection occur in sinuses. These may cause a number of problems including sinusitis or rhinitis, headaches etc. So keeping the sinuses clean and healthy is necessary. This yog kriya does exactly this by using water.

This kriya is popularly known as 'neti'. If it is done with water it is called 'jal neti' and when performed with cotton threads then it is called 'sutra neti'. Jal neti is easier and safer to practise. It is also popularly known as 'nasal irrigation'.

To perform this cleansing kriya you will need a pot especially made for this purpose. It is called 'jal neti pot'. You can procure it from any yoga centre or buy it from Amazon.

How to do it

Fill the 'jal neti pot' with luke warm water. Add some (1/5 table spoon) salt to it. Mix the salt well. Now insert the tip of the tube (coming out of neti pot) in your left nostril. Bend slightly forward and on your right. Start breathing from mouth. Now allow the water from the 'neti pot' to enter your nostril. If everything goes well this water should come out of your right nostril. Keep on breathing from mouth and allow all the water in the pot to enter your left nostril and come out from right nostril. Repeat with opposite nostril.

Key to doing it properly lies in 'breathing from mouth'. While performing this 'kriya', if you use your nostrils for breathing then you won't be able to do it. So before allowing the water to enter into your nostril, start breathing from mouth.

Luke warm water is used to match the temperature of your body and also because it better cleans the nasal passages and sinuses. Little bit of salt is added to water to match the salinity of your body. Furthermore, salt is more effective in removing cough deposited on sinus walls. If you don't put salt into the water, it can be a painful experience and your nostrils may become sore. With the proper temperature of water and proper amount of salt added to it, this 'kriya' becomes very easy, just like a cakewalk.

After performing this 'kriya', bend forward and breathe at a fast pace for a while. Doing so will remove remaining water particles in nostrils and sinuses and thus properly dry it.

This 'kriya' should be done preferably in the morning and never in the evening. If performed in the evening, it can cause cold.

Benefits

This 'kriya' effectively cleans nasal passages and sinuses, thus prevents any infection in it. Some people develop worms in their sinuses. This is a very painful condition. These worms may cause headaches. Even after operations, worms develop time and again. If you keep practicing this kriya, there won't be any such possibility. It is very helpful in treatment of allergic sinusitis. Frequency and intensity of attacks will keep on decreasing and after some time will vanish completely.

This 'kriya' has very beneficial influence on eyes as well as brain. A number of people have been able to leave their 'glasses' (spectacles) by performing this kriya. It has a calming and balancing influence on brain. Tendency to worry on trifles, hypertension, depression, anxiety attacks etc all such problems are relieved by performing this 'kriya'.

Alongwith so many other benefits of this 'kriya', headaches of many types including tension headaches, cluster headaches, headaches due to eye strain, headaches due to sinuses etc just go away. Your body can no more be a refuge for such headaches.

Precautions

This 'kriya' should be done preferably in the morning and never in the evening. If performed in the evening, it can cause cold.

If you are already suffering from infection in sinuses, then before starting practice of this kriya, you should consult your doctor.

If your doctor has prevented you from stooping forward (due to sciatica, or disc bulge etc) then you may not be able to do it.

Bowel irrigation

There is another kriya in yoga which is performed with the help of water. This kriya cleanses bowels. It is called 'basti', also known as bowel irrigation. It cleanses your bowels very well. It cleans and revogorates them. It frees you from constipation and a number of other bowel related problems.

If we eat oily foods and fine grains more often then these stick to the walls of the bowel. Over a period of time this layer thickens. This thickened layer adds weight to the bowels and peristalsis movement of bowels is limited due to this increased weight. Peristalsis movement is basically a wave like motion of bowels through which it pushes its contents down the tract. With the decreased peristalsis movement the problem of constipation further increases. The person falls in a vicious circle. At places such layers are also formed upon undigested food particles in the bowels. With the passage of time layers upon layers accumulate on them and they become hard as stones. They and are termed as 'faecoliths' (stones formed of faeces).

These layers and faecoliths become harbouring ground for bad bacteria which may cause a number of diseases including allergy etc. Bowel irrigation gradually removes these layers and frees one from these faecoliths. Once bowels are cleaned their functionality returns. Peristalsis movement increases. They become more efficient in absorbing nutrients. Clean bowels are also a better place for proper growth of good bacteria. These good bacteria assist the body in the process of digestion. They also synthesize various vitamins needed by the body like Vitamin D and K etc and supply them to the body.

Whenever someone resorts to fasting or decides to decrease his diet or remains on only liquids like juices etc he should and must practice bowel irrigation. Due to decreased volume of food eaten one may suffer from constipation and may not be able to get full benefits of fasting or any specific diet plan. Bowel irrigation addresses this problem.

How to do it and when

It can be done any time of the day but morning hours are the best. To perform bowel irrigation you will need rectal syringes or anema pumps. You can easily buy them from Amazon. Fill the rectal syringe with luke warm water and insert this water into your rectum through rectal syringe. You may apply some oil on the tip of the syringe as well as on the anus, so that it enters smoothly. You should also check for sharp edges at the tip of the rectal syringe, it may cause wounds in your anus. If you find any sharp edges cut and remove them. Take about 1 litre of water inside your rectum. Now squeeze your anus inside and upwards so that water taken inside the rectum goes up into bowel. Now walk for a while. Try to keep this water inside your bowels for about 15 minutes. After you feel pressure, go to toilet. This water will bring out a lot of constipated faeces and other impurities from the bowel along with it. You can add some medicinal value also to this water. Boil some leaves of Neem (Azadiracta Indica) in the water. Take out the leaves and use this water for putting into your rectum once it cools down to lukewarm level. If you cannot get Azadiracta leaves you can use it's oil also which is readily available at Ayurvedic medicine shops. In place of Azadiracta Indica you can also use curcumin or any other medicinal herb. Benefit of adding the properties of Azadiracta Indica in the water that you take inside your bowels is that it will kill worms and bad bacteria there. It will make it very difficult for worms and bad bacteria to make your colon their house. Adding curcumin in the water will help in you getting rid from a number of inflammatory conditions in your body as it has anti-inflammatory property. After practising it for a few days you will feel fresher, lighter, more energetic and more youthful.

Benefits of Bowel Irrigation

Bowel irrigation is recommended for a number of allergies and auto immune diseases like Asthma, Irritable Bowel Syndrome etc. It is supposed that the root cause of allergy and auto immune diseases is some problem with gut flora. Gut flora is a term used for the group of bacteria residing in your colon.

These bacteria help us in many ways. First they check the growth of bad bacteria and aid our body's defense system. They fight from them and keep them at bay. Secondly, if they cannot fight any bad bacteria, they send signals to our immune system to produce antibodies so that these bacteria may not enter our body and even if they enter they can be killed by our body's defense system. At times gut flora sends wrong signals and body's defense system start acting against its own parts. This is what happens in the case of various allergies and auto immune diseases. Bowel irrigation addresses this problem. It has positive impact on gut flora and can make them friendlier to our body.

It frees you from constipation. Cleanses the walls of colon and make them more efficient. Furthermore, your body can absorb water from your colon also. Thus it also helps in hydrating your body. It is very effective in maintaining high level of hydration in the body.

Kunjal Kriya

Kunjal Kriya or Kunjar Kriya or Vyaghra Kriya is basically a detoxification process used in yoga. It has many benefits. First, it clears all the mucus and other impurities in the throat and thus gives relief in Asthma, chronic cough etc. Secondly, it cleans the stomach. It removes excess acids, undigested food items, bile etc from the stomach. By cleaning the stomach it strengthens the digestion. Third and *most importantly, it throws out pent up emotions from the stomach, the task which cannot be done by any other means.* Actually, in present day world, all of us have some negative emotions which we cannot take out safely. Boss has chided you in the office. You cannot give befitting reply to your boss. Your anger towards your boss has got deposited in your body. Your wife is misbehaving with you but you cannot tell it to anyone else due to the fear that they will make fun of you. This negative emotion has also got deposited into your body. All such negative emotions get deposited in your stomach. When you perform this kriya, water brings out these negative emotions also along with it. As a result, you will feel lighter and more refreshed. Clearly discernible impact will be seen on your mood and health.

How to do it

Sit in squatting position, as if you are sitting on a squatty toilet. Drink 5-6 glasses of water at a fast pace. Once you feel that you cannot drink any more water and feel nauseated, stand up. Lean a bit forward and insert your index and middle finger in your mouth and press the base of your tongue. Doing so will induce vomiting. Vomit all the water that you have just taken in. Initially only plain water will come out, but later on acidic water, bile, undigested food particles etc may come out. It is better to use luke warm water for this. Though, yoga scriptures ask you to add some salt to this water, but I don't suggest it, because for many of you it may difficult to vomit all the water out. Any salty water that remains in your body will adversely affect your health. You can repeat this process twice or thrice in one sitting, as for most of you first time may not be enough to properly clean your stomach. Some of you may need to take 10-12 glasses of water or even more to reach a nauseating state. Though it needs some will power to do it, but believe me it is worth it. You don't need to do it every day. Even once a week will do. During acute Asthma attacks or chronic cough, you may want to do it continually for a week.

Precautions

If you have any heart problem or are suffering from any serious problem of stomach then you should not do it. Though, it is harmless, it is better to try it for the first time under the guidance of an experienced yoga teacher.

You should any take anything (even liquid or water) upto 30 minutes of doing this kriya.

Steam bath

Many of might have taken 'steam bath' or 'sauna bath' or at least have planned to take it at some point of time in future. Steam bath is another way to purify body. It opens the pores of the skin and throws out toxins from the body. However, if you don't properly prepare your body for taking sauna bath, in place of benefiting from it, you may become dehydrated and fall ill.

Preparations for taking steam bath

During sauna bath or steam bath you will perspire profusely and your body will lose water as crazy. So you must take enough luke warm water before entering into sauna room. This water will keep you hydrated even after profuse sweating. You should also keep a wet towel on your head. It will save your brain from heating and keep it cool. Literally, it is very necessary to keep your head cool.

How to reap maximum benefit from sauna bath

In order to reap maximum benefit from sauna bath you should massage your full body with oil and leave the oil for about half an hour before entering into sauna room. Oil enters deep into the skin pores and attaches various impurities and toxins with itself. When one takes steam bath, oil comes out with sweat and also brings out the impurities along with it. Thus better flushing out of toxins from the body occurs.

What to do after coming out of sauna room

After coming out of sauna bath one should take bath with warm water. If you take bath with cold water or water at room temperature, your body will have to cope with sudden change in temperature and you may fall ill. As during steam bath a lot of water and electrolytes are lost by the body, you should also take ORS after coming out of it, so that electrolyte balance in the body may be restored.

More beneficial after oil massage taking luke warm water Before taking steam bath

Kati snan

Water cure for various diseases

Asthma

Asthma can be due to a number of reasons. First and foremost is allergy. Whenever a person is exposed to allergens, allergic reactions start in the body, Mucus is formed in alveoli of lungs and internal walls of trachea become inflamed and constricted leading to dyspnoea and choking of breath. Due to indigestion and gastritis also when abdomen is bloated one may feel difficulty in breathing. Bloating puts pressure on heart and interferes in normal functioning of heart. Due to improper functioning of heart, one feels problems in breathing. When one feels problems in breathing, cough is deposited in trachea (tube through which air passes before entering into lungs), which further aggravates breathing problem. This is called cardiac cough.

Water cure is very effective in treatment of Asthma. Whatever be the reason of Asthma, water cure works miraculously and significantly decreases the intensity as well as frequency i.e. subsequent Asthama attacks will be increasingly less violent and on longer intervals.

Water cure strategy for Asthma

Water cure strategy for Asthma has three elements i.e. (i) drink warm water, (ii) practise kunjar kriya and (iii) bowel irrigation frequently. At the time of attack or otherwise also always try to drink luke warm water. During the time of attack, Kunjar kriya can be practised daily. Otherwise once or twice a week should suffice. Similarly bowel irrigation should be practised at least once a week, preferably twice a week. Preferably you should boil the water along with neem (Azadiracta Indica) leaves and let it cool down to lukewarm level before using it for bowel irrigation. If you follow this regime, very soon you will notice that attacks of Asthma have decreased significantly in intensity as well as frequency.

Another important point to note is that all efforts should be made to avoid constipation. Avoiding constipation doesn't mean that you start taking laxatives. Laxatives are a strict 'no no' for Asthmatic patients and should be avoided at all costs. They cause dehydration in the body in general and in vital organs in particular. Do you know how laxatives work? When you take laxatives, once it reaches large intestine, it soaks water from the body through walls of large intestine. This water then makes the stool soft so that it can be easily evacuated from the body. No doubt you pass stool easily in the morning after taking laxative, but you lose significant amount of water, minerals and precious electrolytes during the process that too from your vital organs. What do you think, which organs will supply this water to large intestine? Only nearby organs can supply this water. Which organs are nearby to large intestine? Small intestine, stomach, liver and Kidneys, all these key and vital organs are located near large intestine. So, definitely all this water is coming from these organs. After losing water, there is bound to be a drop in the efficiency of these organs. Can you hope to remain healthy after losing so much water and nutrients from your body's key and vital organs? In normal conditions, it is the large intestine which acts as an extra water bag for the body from where body can take water in times of need. But laxatives reverse the process. Body is losing water to the organ from where it could have taken it. Due to this very reason laxatives are bound to make you ill, severely ill, after a period of time. The job that laxatives does should be done by dietary fiber. If you take sufficient amount of dietary fiber they you will not laxatives. Dietary fibers absorb water and keep them trapped in them. When these fiber reach large intestine there is sufficient water in the large intestine both for making stools soft and for supplying to the body in times of need, all thanks to fibers. This is the best natural process which you should try to ensure that your body follows. However, if for some or the other reason you have to take laxatives and it cannot be avoided, then after taking laxative you should drink sufficient amount of water, so that your body doesn't feel shortage of water even after losing it in significant amounts to your large intestine.

How luke warm water helps in Asthma

Luke warm water helps at many levels. First it aids digestion. Digestive processes become more efficient with it. With improved digestion, less toxins are produced in the body and the load on your liver decreases. Process of digestion can be compared with fire. If there is proper fire, fuels burn properly and less smoke is produced. If there is not proper fire, fuels don't burn properly and large amount of smoke is produced. In this simily, fire is your digestion process, fuel is the food you take and smoke is the toxins that are produced as a by product of digestion. In fact fire and fuel are co-dependent upon each other. If fuel is of good quality, it is easier to make fire and the fuel burns properly. On the other hand if fire is big and proper, even poor quality fuels burn well. Similar is the condition with your digestion. If you take easily digestible food then there will be proper digestion and less toxins will be produced. However, if your digestion power is strong, even 'tough to digest food' are digested well and less toxins are produced. Secondly, it increases body heat. When you drink luke warm water, your body cools it down to the level of body temperature before using it. In the process your body gains some heat. Heat is also gained by your body when there is proper digestion of food. Third, it is easier for your body to absorb and assimilate luke warm water. It is easily used by the body at cellular level.

Due to all these benefits drinking luke warm water helps immensely in Asthma. During Asthma attacks one should drink only luke warm water and eat easily digestible food.

How Kunjar Kriya helps in Asthma

Kunjar kriya helps in improving digestion as well as removes cough deposited in trachea and lungs. Once dried cough is expelled from trachea and lungs, intensity and frequency of Asthma attacks automatically decrease. Kunjar kriya also releases pent up emotions which may be the prime reason in significant number of cases of Asthma. It also stimulates internal walls of trachea and makes them healthier. Healthier internal walls of trachea literally means lessened intensity and frequency of Asthma attacks. While performing kunjar kriya when you press in the backward portion of tongue you are stimulating Vishuddhi Chakra. As per yoga scriptures, Asthma is a disease caused by malfunction of Vishuddhi chakra which is responsible for detoxification of the body. Once Vishuddhi Chakra is stimulated you get definite relief in Asthma. This kriya also stimulates Manipur chakra which is responsible for proper digestion and heat in the body. As per Ayurvedic principles, Asthma is a disease caused by decrease in body heat. It is a truth that invariably in all Asthma patients you will find decreased body heat, poor digestion, poor function of liver, increased toxicity in the body etc. This kriya helps on all these fronts.

How bowel irrigation helps in Asthma

Bowel irrigation helps in Asthma at various levels. First it improves the quality of gut flora. All the worms and bad bacteria are evacuated from large intestine by bowel irrigation. All types of allergies have origin in some abnormalities in gut flora. Once proper balance is established in gut flora allergies decrease. Secondly, it helps relieve constipation and faecoliths. It also stimulates Muladhar chakra, Swadhisthan Chakra and Manipur Chakra. Muladhar Chakra is directly associated with strength in the body. Once Muladhar Chakra is stimulated it strengthens the whole body. With the increased strength in the body, Asthma is gradually cured. Swadhisthan chakra is responsible for regulation of water in the body. With the stimulation of

Swadhisthan Chakra water is used in more efficient ways in the body and the problem of cough is lessened significantly as it will be formed only when and where it is necessary (cough has significant amount of water content) and also there will be only as much water in the cough as is optimum. There will be no problem of either dried cough or excessive cough in the body. Manipur chakra is responsible for proper digestion and body heat. With the stimulation of Manipur chakra, digestion improves and body heat increases. All excess cough is burnt by Manipur chakra.

Acidity, acid reflux, heart burn and indigestion

Water cure is very effective in curing acidity, acid reflux and indigestion.

Strategy for treatment of acidity, acid reflux and indigestion has three elements (i) drink warm water, (ii) practise Kunjar Kriya and (iii) Bowel irrigation.

Drink one glass (about 200 ml) of luke warm water 30 minutes before taking meal. It will prepare your stomach and digestive system for digestion of meal. Don't eat water during meal. Drink one glass of luke warm water after 30 minutes of taking meal. Drink one liter of luke warm water after three hours of taking meal. Following this regime will strengthen your digestive system and ensure proper digestion of meal taken.

Kunjar Kriya can be practised when you are suffering from acidity any time of the day. It will relieve you from severest of acidity immediately. You may need to perform it twice or thrice in one sitting. One set of vomiting is count one. After one set of vomiting, again drink water to full and vomit. This will be count two. You may need to repeat this kriya upto the count of three. Don't take anything (even water) upto 30 minutes after performing this kriya. This kriya cleanses the stomach and removes all the toxins and unevacuated waste from it. Thus, it strengthens your digestion power. All the acid is thrown out by this kriya so you get immediate relief in severest of acidity. As undigested food items are also thrown out, the root cause of your acidity, acid reflux and heart burn is removed.

Bowel irrigation should also be practised at least once a week, preferably twice a week. It will strengthen your digestive power. You should add properties of neem in the water to be used for bowel irrigation. Do read topic on bowel irigation under the chapter for Asthma.

You should also keep in mind that for getting rid from acidity, acid reflux etc you should keep in check intake of tea, coffee, cold drinks, soft drinks, sugary drinks, processed food, too fried and spciy food etc. All of them cause acidity and will worsen your problem. Instead you should take easily digestible meals.

You should take your dinner (night meal) at least two hours before going to bed. It will give time to your dinner to be digested. If possible walk for a while after taking your dinner.

Acne

Acne can be due to various reasons. Most imporatant and frequent among them are hormonal changes and constipation. Another major cause of acne is malfunctioing or inefficiency of liver. Liver is the most powerful detoxifier in our body. When it malfunctions or becomes less efficient detoxification process in the process is adversely affected. When toxins accumulate at cellular level they throw them out and these toxins are carried by our lymphatic system to skins to be thrown out through skin. Your acnes are nothing else but miniscules bags containing toxins mixed with lymphatic fluid of body. Low level of hydration aids acne to appear and makes it severe.

Once hydration level in your body increases, liver starts functioning properly and there is no constipation, your acnes will vanish on their own.

During puberty when hormonal changes occur in the body at a very fast pace, acnes are normal to appear. Second time such phase comes in the life of a woman is during menopause.

In 99 percent of cases water cure alone can completely free you from acne and gift you a healthy glowing skin naturally. You don't need any cream, moisturiser or medicine.

Water cure strategy for treatment of acne has mainly two elements (i) drink warm water and (ii) bowel irrigation.

Start your day by drinking as much warm water as you can drink without nauseating. Include sufficient amount of dietary fiber in your diet. This is an essential element of water cure and is necessary for increasing your hydration level.

Besides above, drink one glass (about 200 ml) of luke warm water 30 minutes before taking meal. It will prepare your stomach and digestive system for digestion of meal. Don't eat water during meal. Drink one glass of luke warm water after 30 minutes of taking meal. Drink one liter of luke warm water after three hours of taking meal. Following this regime will strengthen your digestive system and ensure proper digestion of meal taken. Proper digestion of food literally means less toxicity and lesser load on liver.

Bowel irigation increases hydration level in the body very efficiently. They also free you from constipation another frequent and significant cause of constipation. You should practise bowel irrigation at least thrice a week. you should add properties of neem in the water to be used for bowel irrigation. Do read topic on bowel irigation under the chapter for Asthma.

Constipation

Constipation is the root cause of many diseases. As a number of waster materials of the body can be reabsorbed by the body through large intestinge, constipation increases toxicity in the body. Direct impact is on digestion and skin. With increased toxicity in the body load on liver increases. As a result of excessive load, efficiency of liver may decrease or it may start malfunctioning altogether. This further aggravates the situation. Gradually a number of disease make their home in your body.

Water cure is most effective in the treatment of constipation. Toughest of constipation can be completely cured by water cure.

Water cure strategy for the treatment has mainly one element i.e. bowel irrigation. Practise it at least thrice a week. Intially you may like to do it daily. It will cure your constipation and increase hydration level in the body.

Besides practising bowel irrigation you should also drink warm water. Start your day by drinking as much warm water as you can drink without nauseating. The moment warm water reaches your colon it relaxes smooth muscles there large intestine springs into action to throw out accumulated waste material.

Also include sufficient amount of dietary fiber in your diet. This is an essential element of water cure and is necessary for increasing your hydration level.

Besides above, drink one glass (about 200 ml) of luke warm water 30 minutes before taking meal. It will prepare your stomach and digestive system for digestion of meal. Don't eat water during meal. Drink one glass of luke warm water after 30 minutes of taking meal. Drink one liter of luke warm water after three hours of taking meal. Following this regime will strengthen your digestive system and ensure proper digestion of meal taken. Proper digestion of food literally means less toxicity and lesser load on liver.

Diabetes

Diabetes is basically a result of chronic indigestion and acidity. Pancreas whose Beta cells secretes insulin and in the case of diabetes stops secreting it has another role also. It secretes bi-carbonate in order to neutralise the acidity of the stomach. If someone suffers continuously from acidity, pancreas is over burdened and its other functionalities including secretion of insulin by its beta cells is decreased. Down the course of time diabetes develops. Thus in order to reverse diabetes one needs to strengthen his digestive system and control acidity. By controlling indigestion and acidity one can reverse the process of diabetes. If its beta cells has not suffered reversible damage then they can be revived by controlling acidity and indigetion.

Read the previous chapter on acidity and indigestion. Additionally, bowel irrigation has been found very effective in controlling diabetes. **While treating diabetes through water cure you need to focus more on bowel irrigation. It should be performed at least thrice a week.** By adopting the techniques of water cure your dependency on diabetes medicines will gradually decrease and if you are lucky (no irreversible damage has been made to beta cells of pancreas), your diabetes can be cured completely.

Start your day by drinking as much water as you can drink without nauseating. Include sufficient amount of dietary fiber in your diet. This is an essential element of water cure and is necessary for increasing your hydration level. Do read the chpater 'when and how much water to drink'.

Cardiovascular and Heart diseases

Water cure basically helps in cardiovasclar and heart diseases by removing cholesterol from arteries and veins. Basically, water cure improves the functioning of liver. When functioning of liver improves it takes out cholesterol from blood and uses it in production of fresh bile. This fresh bile is used for digestion of fat. Thus it helps in two ways. First it ensures proper digestion of fat by secreting more fresh bile. Secondly, it removes extra cholesterol from the blood, thus gradually cholesterol plaques in arteries and veins are removed thereby ensuring uninterrupted and smooth flow of blood through them. Once smooth and uniterrupted flow of blood through arteries and veins is ensured, load on heart decreases and its functioning improves.

Furthermore, once level of hydration in the body increases through water cure, elasticity of walls of arteries and veins are also restored, which in turn further improves the functioning of heart.

With improved digestion gastritis also remains in control. In a number of cases of heart problems, basically bloated stomach puts pressure on diaphragm which make breathing difficult and this difficult breathing puts extra load on heart giving rise to heart problems. With relief in gastritis, this burden on heart is removed.

All cardiovascular and heart diseases including angina pain, atherosclersis, arythima, palpitation, dysponea etc gradually vanish.

Start your day with taking as much of luke warm water as you can drink without nauseating and do walk at comfortable pace for at least 30 minutes. Include sufficient amount of dietary fiber in your diet. This is an essential element of water cure and is necessary for increasing your hydration level. Do read the chpater 'when and how much water to drink'.

If your suffering from heart disease or high blood pressure you should not practise kunjar kriya, I repeat DO NOT PRACTISE KUNJAR KRIYA IF YOU ARE SUFFERING FROM HEART DISEASE OR HIGH BLOOD PRESSURE.

Practise bowel irrigation at least twice a week.

Do read chapter on indigestion, acidity etc and Asthma.

Arthritis, joint pain, knee pain and back pain

Water cure helps in arthritis and joint pains (including knee pain and back pain) by ensuring proper water content in synovial and cerebrospinal fluid. Once the level of hydration increases in the body, sufficient water is available in the body for adding to synovial fluid and cerebrospinal fluid. If you are lucky (irreversible damages have not been made on cartilages and joints) your arthritis, joints pain, knee pain and back pain can be completely cured. With sufficient water in synovial fluid and crebrospinal fluid proper nutrition of cartilages in the joints and vertebrae (carliages in between two vertebrae is called disc) is ensured. So they are better able to recover from injuries and day to day wear and tear.

Start your day with taking as much of luke warm water as you can drink without nauseating. Include sufficient amount of dietary fiber in your diet. This is an essential element of water cure and is necessary for increasing your hydration level. Do read the chpater 'when and how much water to drink'.

Kunjar Kriya is not necessary but bowel irrigation should be practised at least twice a week.

Skin diseases: get healthy glowing skin naturally

With increased hydration in the body moisture in the skin cells increase. Increased hydration also ensures proper detoxification of skin cells and tissues as well as whole body. With improvement in digestion and functioning of liver detoxification process in the body also become efficient. As a combined effect of all these factors you get healthy glowing skin naturally. With increased hydration all skin disease gradually vanish.

At times skin disease may be due to blocked skin pores. Steam bath is very good for such cases.

Start your day with taking as much luke warm water as you can drink without nauseating. Include sufficient amount of dietary fiber in your diet. This is an essential element of water cure and is necessary for increasing your hydration level. Do read the chpater 'when and how much water to drink'.

Obesity: get clearly discernible results within four weeks

Obesity is basically a problem of improper digestion. Due to inefficient digestion process, body is unable to extract proper amount of nutrients from the food. In order to compensate for this lack brain creates cravings for food and by eating more food one becomes obese.

Water cure is very effective in curing obesity. By improving digestion, it ensures proper digestion and assimilation of fat so it doesn't get deposited in the body. Instead fat is used up by the body efficiently. With decreased amount of deposited fat in the body obesity decreases significantly very soon. It gives clearly discerinble results within four weeks.

Start your day with taking as much water as you can drink wihtout nauseating. Always drink luke warm water. Practise bowel irrigation at least thrice a week. Include sufficient amount of dietary fiber in your diet. This is an essential element of water cure and is necessary for increasing your hydration level. Do read the chpater 'when and how much water to drink'.

Erectile Dysfunction

Water cure helps significantly in curing erectile dysfunction, esepcially bowel irrigation. It stimulates Muladhar chakra which controls sexual power. With the stimulation of Muladhar chakra, sexual power increases. All those suffering with erectile dysfunction should must practise bowel irrigation at least thrice a weak. It also relaxes the smooth muscles in pelvic area thereby increasing blood flow to penis. Do read topic on bowel irrigation in the chapter on Asthma.

For more information on erectile dysfunction and its natural cure you can read the book 'How to ge rid of Erectile Dysfunction naturally' by Rajat Sharma.

Kidney stone and Kidney pain

Formation of stones in kidneys is basically due to low water level and increased acidity in the body. It is basically a symptom of chronic dehydration. Whenever water level decreases in the body acidity in the body increases. Brain instructs kidneys to extract less water from the blood and make less urine. As urine is lesser in amount concentration of waste materials in it increases. Its density as well as acidity both increases. As there are more waste materials in the urine and water content is less, waster materials start depositing in kidney. With the passage of time layers above layers of wastes form upon these deposited wastes, which finally take the form of stones. Whenever these stones get trapped in the walls of kidneys, or ureter or urethra while coming out from there, they cause unbearable pain. This is called Kidney pain.

In most of the cases, especially when kidney stones are smaller in size, drinking one litre of water immediately relieves kidney pain. Once water level in the body increases, brain instructs kidneys to extract more water from the blood and make more urine, as soon as volume of urine and amount of water in it increases, these smaller stones are passed through urethra easily. However, if size of Kidney stone is large it may need to be broken first either through medicine, or laser or laproscopic surgery. In extreme cases, surgery may be needed to remove them.

Prevention is better than cure. So it is better to not let the stone being formed in Kidneys. If you maintain adequate hydration level in the body, no stones will be formed and in majority of the cases even already formed stones will be gradually thrown out of the body along with urine.

Start your day with drinking as much of luke water water as you can drink without nauseating. Include sufficient amount of dietary fiber in your diet. This is an essential element of water cure and is necessary for increasing your hydration level. Do read the chpater 'when and how much water to drink'.

You may not need any advanced method of water cure for getting rid from Kidney pain. However, you should practise bowel irrigation at least once a week. These are very effective in increasing hydration level in the body.

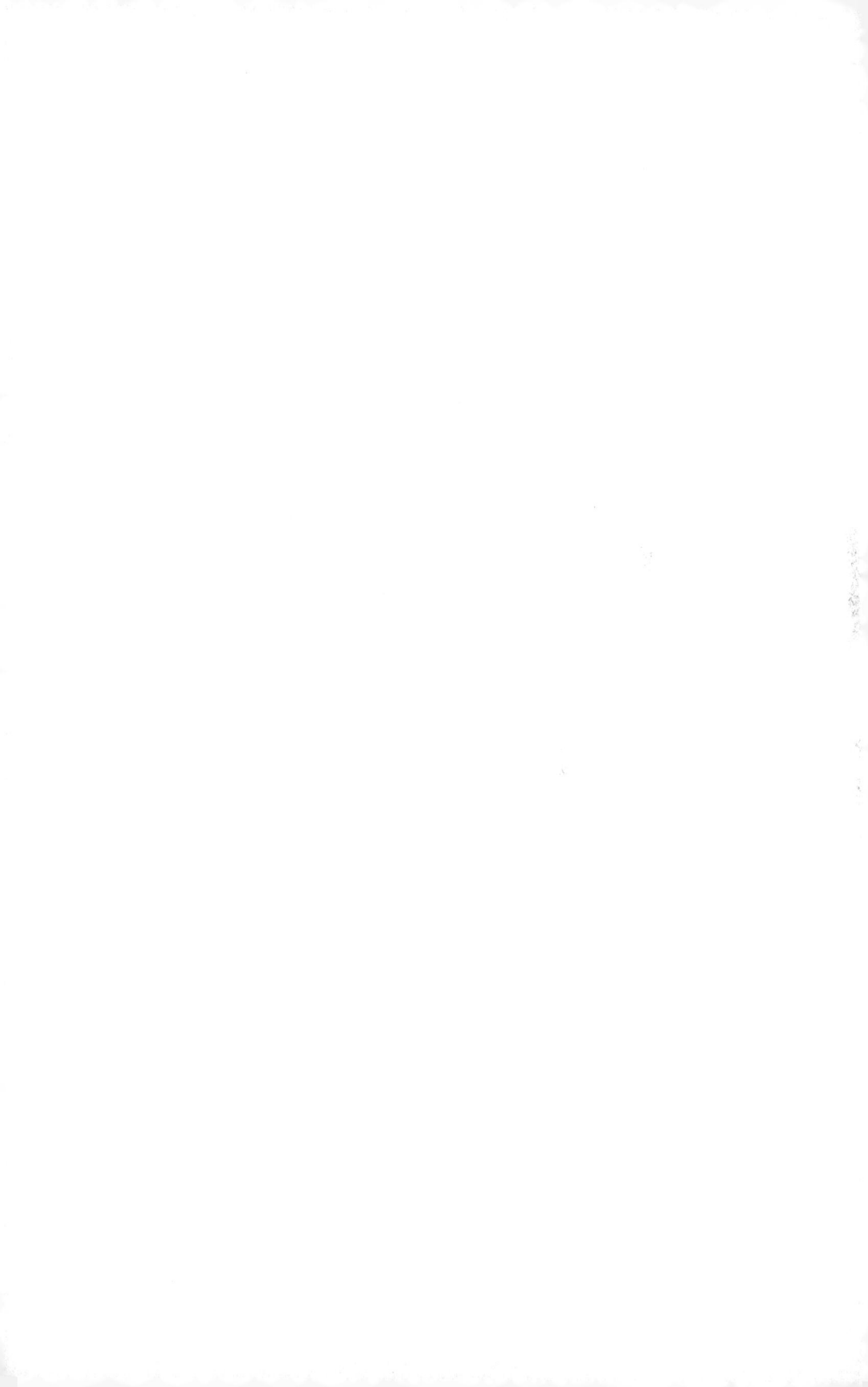

Scaly and dried lips

Scaly, dried and cracked lips are basically indicators of low level of hydration in the body. Once hydration level increases in the body through water cure, your lips will become soft and supple.

Start your day with drinking as much of luke warm water as you can drink without nauseating. Include sufficient amount of dietary fiber in your diet. This is an essential element of water cure and is necessary for increasing your hydration level. Do read the chpater 'when and how much water to drink'.

Hair fall

Hair fall can be due to various reasons including genetics, hormonal changes, anaemia and low hydration level in the body. Deficiency of some minerals like Selenium and Zinc also cause hair fall. You can take Zinc and Selenium supplements to address deficiency of these minerals. Poor blood circulation is also one of the reasons of hair fall. Due to poor blood circulation, hair roots don't get sufficient nutrients and become weak. In order to improve blood circulation in your body you should do aerobic exercises for at least 10 minutes every day. With the low level of hydration in the body hair roots become drier and weaker.

Start your day with drinking as much of luke warm water as you can drink without nauseating. Include sufficient amount of dietary fiber in your diet. This is an essential element of water cure and is necessary for increasing your hydration level. Do read the chpater 'when and how much water to drink'.

You don't need any advanced method of water cure. However, you can practise bowel irrigation twice a week. Bowel irrigation is very effective in increasing hydration level in the body.

Headache

Water cure is very effective in curing headache. It may not give immediate relief but works wonderfully in cases of chronic headaches.

With increased hydration level in the body, cardio vascular system become healthier and more efficient (read chapter on heart diseases) thus headaches due to high blood pressure or blockages in arteries and veins gradually vanish.

Another major cause of headache is blockages, inflammations or infections in sinuses. Water cure is very effective in cleansing sinuses and treatment of blockages, inflammations and infections in sinuses.

Practise nasal irrigation or jal neti at least thrice a week. It will cure all the problems related with sinuses. With the improvement in health of sinuses, your headache will go away like a magic. If you have severe and chronic infections in sinuses consult your doctor before practising nasal irrigation.

Start your day with drinking as much of luke warm water as you can drink without nauseating. Include sufficient amount of dietary fiber in your diet. This is an essential element of water cure and is necessary for increasing your hydration level. Do read the chpater 'when and how much water to drink'

For more information on headaches you can read my book titled 'How to get instant releif from headache instantly'. By following the techniques told in this book you can get instant relife in most types of headaches that too without taking any medicine.

Sinusitis/Rhinitis

Water cure is very effective in treatment of sinusitis and rhinitis. During the attacks of sinsitis and rhinitis drink only luke warm water.

Practise nasal irrigation or jal neti at least thrice a week. It will cure all the problems related with sinuses. If you have severe and chronic infections in sinuses consult your doctor before practising nasal irrigation.

If the cause of your sinusitis or rhinitis is allergy, you should practise bowel irrigation at least thrice a week. Bowel irrigation is very effective in curing allergy. It will gradually decrease your allergic reactions and over a period of time will bring them down to negligible levels.

Conclusion

I hope you have enjoyed reading my book. It would have enlightened you upon significance of water, benefits of drinking it, its role in the body, necessity of water cure etc. It would have also apprised you of various advanced methods of water cure.

If you liked reading this book. You may like to read my other books also.

How to get rid of Sciatica and lower back pain without exercises

&

How to get instant relief from headache

If you have any suggestion or complaint you can write to me at bhaskarmishra883@gmail.com

With best wishes

Yours Bhaskar Mishra

Printed in Great Britain
by Amazon